Beating Epilepsy

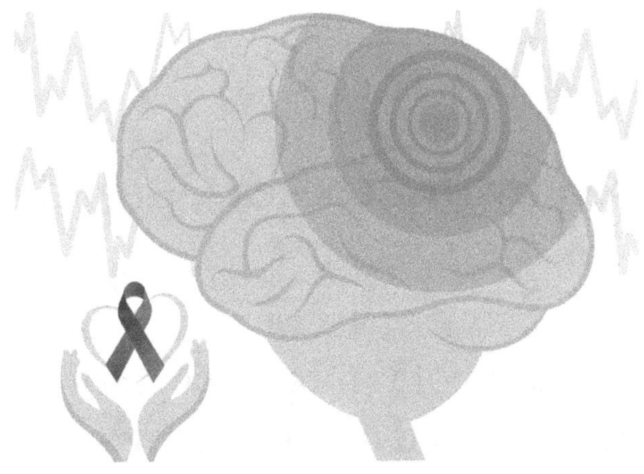

A Comprehensive Guide For Living Well With Epilepsy For Newly Diagnosed Patient And Caregiver.

Rebecca J. Reynolds

Content

INTRODUCTION

The moment a diagnosis of epilepsy is delivered, it can be likened to an unexpected tempest that sweeps over your life. A sudden onslaught of uncertainty, fear, and a myriad of questions envelops you, leaving both you and your loved ones grappling for explanations.

In the face of this tumultuous experience, "Beating Epilepsy: A Comprehensive Guide for Living Well with Epilepsy for Newly Diagnosed Patients and Caregivers" emerges as your steadfast beacon. Envision a lighthouse standing tall against the storm. Its robust beam pierces through the darkness, guiding ships safely to harbor. This book assumes that role, casting a luminous glow on the path that lies ahead. It doesn't merely provide information; it becomes your guiding light, arming you with the knowledge and tools essential to navigate the intricate landscape of epilepsy and lead a gratifying life despite the inherent challenges.

Whether you find yourself at the center of the diagnosis or standing in solidarity with someone who is, this book evolves into your unwavering companion. Within its pages, a treasure trove of insights awaits:

Detailed elucidations on epilepsy, encompassing its various types, causes, and treatment options. By demystifying medical terminology, it aids in comprehending the condition, facilitating informed decisions about your healthcare.
Pragmatic counsel on seizure management, ranging from medication regimens to adjustments in lifestyle. It unveils effective strategies to diminish both the frequency and severity of seizures.
Coping mechanisms designed to nurture emotional well-being. It addresses the prevalent anxiety, depression, and societal stigma often intertwined with epilepsy, fostering resilience and empowerment.
A plethora of resources and support networks that establish connections with invaluable organizations, communities, and healthcare professionals capable of offering guidance and encouragement.

"Beating Epilepsy" transcends the boundaries of being a mere book; it transforms into a lifeline. It assembles a community of understanding, serves as a wellspring of hope, and outlines a roadmap towards a life brimming with possibilities.

Turn the page, immerse yourself in the light it offers, and embark on your journey to conquer epilepsy. Together, let us navigate this storm and traverse towards the serene waters that lie beyond.

Real-life Triumphs Over Epilepsy

In the peaceful community of Serenityville, where the promise of hope often struggled to be heard amidst life's uncertainties, a young man named Luke resided. Luke's world took an unforeseen turn when he was confronted with the diagnosis of epilepsy, a turbulent force that cast a shadow over his once tranquil existence.

A climate of uncertainty, fear, and myriad questions enveloped Luke and his family, posing a threat to the light that had previously illuminated their days. It was at this pivotal moment that Luke chanced upon a source of support—the book "Beating Epilepsy." Like a lighthouse emerging from the mist, it served as his guiding beacon, illuminating a path toward resilience and triumph.

Luke immersed himself in the pages of this comprehensive guide, discovering more than mere information; it provided him with a roadmap to navigate the intricacies of epilepsy. The lucid explanations demystified the medical terminology, empowering Luke to make informed decisions about his healthcare. The practical guidance on seizure management acted as his guiding compass, leading him through medication regimens and lifestyle adjustments that gradually alleviated the frequency and severity of his episodes.

However, the journey was not solely about managing the medical aspects. Luke unearthed a wealth of coping mechanisms for emotional well-being within the book. Confronting the anxiety, depression, and societal stigma often associated with epilepsy, he found the resilience to not just endure but thrive in the face of challenges.

As Luke embarked on this transformative odyssey, the book unfolded into more than a source of information; it evolved into a community of understanding. Luke connected with support networks, invaluable organizations, and compassionate healthcare professionals who stood by his side. The initial isolation he experienced transformed into a sense of belonging, and the collective strength of the community became a formidable force against the storms of epilepsy.

Armed with newfound hope and knowledge, Luke turned the pages, stepped into the light, and began crafting his narrative of victory over epilepsy. Serenity gradually returned to Serenityville, not as

an absence of challenges but as the tranquil waters
beyond the storm.

Today, Luke's story resonates throughout the town,
serving as an inspiration for those facing similar
challenges. His triumph stands as proof of the
transformative power of resilience, community, and
the guidance found within the pages of "Beating
Epilepsy." In Serenityville, hope endures, and
Luke's journey remains a guiding light for those
navigating their storms, reminding them that victory
is not only conceivable but within their grasp.

Dear Buyers of "Beating Epilepsy

 extends its embrace to a diverse audience, recognizing the nuanced challenges faced by individuals navigating the landscape of epilepsy. This invaluable resource is tailored for:

1. Newly Diagnosed Patients: For those who have recently received an epilepsy diagnosis, this book serves as a compass, offering clear explanations to demystify the medical jargon and providing a roadmap for understanding the condition. It becomes a trusted companion, empowering individuals to make informed decisions about their healthcare.

2. Caregivers and Loved Ones: Understanding and supporting someone with epilepsy can be challenging. "Beating Epilepsy" offers insights and guidance for caregivers, equipping them with the tools to provide meaningful support. It addresses not only the medical aspects but also delves into coping mechanisms for emotional well-being, fostering a holistic approach to caregiving.

3. Individuals Managing Seizures: The book provides practical guidance for managing seizures, encompassing medication regimens and lifestyle adjustments. It becomes a valuable resource, offering effective strategies to reduce the frequency and severity of seizures, thereby enhancing the quality of life for those actively managing this aspect of epilepsy.

4.Those Navigating Emotional Challenges: Epilepsy often brings emotional burdens such as anxiety, depression, and societal stigma. "Beating Epilepsy" is a source of empowerment, offering coping mechanisms to address these challenges and encouraging individuals to build resilience, fostering emotional well-being.

5. Community Seekers: Beyond being a book, "Beating Epilepsy" transforms into a community of understanding. It connects readers with support networks, organizations, and healthcare professionals, creating a sense of belonging. This inclusive approach recognizes that facing epilepsy is not a solitary journey but one that can be shared and supported within a community.

6.Healthcare Professionals: The book acts as a valuable resource for healthcare professionals involved in the care of individuals with epilepsy. It provides up-to-date information, insights, and practical advice that can complement medical expertise, facilitating a collaborative approach to patient care.

"Beating Epilepsy" transcends its pages to reach a broad spectrum of individuals affected by epilepsy, offering tailored guidance and support. Whether you are directly managing the condition, caring for someone with epilepsy, or seeking to understand and support the epilepsy community, this comprehensive guide stands as a beacon of knowledge, hope, and resilience.

Part 1: Understanding Epilepsy

Chapter 1

Introduction to Epilepsy

What is epilepsy

Picture your brain as a lively metropolis, teeming with electrical signals facilitating communication across its various sectors. Under normal circumstances, these signals maintain a seamless flow, ensuring everything operates in perfect coordination. However, in epilepsy, it's akin to an abrupt traffic congestion on specific communication pathways.

Epilepsy, put simply, occurs when irregular electrical bursts disrupt the smooth traffic flow in your brain. This sudden surge interrupts the city's usual rhythm, resulting in what we identify as seizures. It's analogous to a short circuit, triggering temporary chaos in different brain regions, contingent on where the congestion occurs.

Envision a seizure as a transient storm impacting the city. Some storms may be fleeting and inconspicuous, resembling a momentary lapse of concentration or a minor muscle twitch. Conversely, others can manifest as intense hurricanes, inducing shaking, loss of consciousness, or peculiar sensations.

While anyone might experience an occasional seizure triggered by factors like a high fever, low blood sugar, or a significant head injury, epilepsy differs. It's comparable to residing in a city susceptible to these electrical storm-seizures, with a heightened likelihood of them recurring without an evident cause.

Dispelling myths and misconceptions

Living with epilepsy can be challenging, and unfortunately, the journey is often burdened by misunderstandings and myths. Here are ten common misconceptions people with epilepsy face, along with the facts to dispel them:

Myth 1: Epilepsy is contagious.

Fact: No, it's not! Epilepsy is a neurological disorder caused by abnormal electrical activity in the brain. You cannot "catch" it through touch or proximity.

Myth 2: All seizures are the same.

Fact: Seizures come in a wide variety, ranging from brief staring spells to convulsions. Their symptoms and types differ based on the brain region affected.

Myth 3: Epilepsy is caused by mental illness.

Fact: Epilepsy is a neurological condition, not a mental illness. While seizures can sometimes affect personality or behavior, they're not a sign of mental instability.

Myth 4: People with epilepsy can't hold jobs or drive.

Fact: With proper medication and seizure control, many people with epilepsy lead fulfilling lives, including holding jobs and driving. Restrictions may vary depending on individual cases and local regulations.

Myth 5: You can swallow someone's tongue during a seizure.

Fact: This is dangerous and unnecessary. During a seizure, people's jaw muscles are usually clenched, making swallowing impossible. Focus on ensuring their safety and waiting for the seizure to pass.

Myth 6: You should restrain someone having a seizure.

Fact: Resisting movement can worsen the seizure. Gently clear the area of hazards and allow the person to recover. Unless they're choking or in immediate danger, avoid holding them down.

Myth 7: Women with epilepsy can't have children.

Fact: Most women with epilepsy can have healthy pregnancies with proper medical supervision. Medications may need adjustments, but it's not a barrier to motherhood.

Myth 8: Epilepsy is a lifelong sentence.

Fact: While some forms are chronic, many people achieve seizure control or even remission through medication and other interventions. Don't lose hope!

Myth 9: People with epilepsy are faking their seizures.

Fact: This is incredibly insensitive and untrue. Seizures are involuntary and a real medical condition. Never question someone's experience based on such assumptions.

Myth 10: Talking about epilepsy is taboo.

Who is affected by epilepsy

Epilepsy is a surprisingly common condition, with an estimated 50 million people living with epilepsy worldwide. That means around 1 in 100 people have epilepsy.

While anyone can develop epilepsy at any point in their life, there are certain groups who are at higher risk:

Age:

Newborns and infants: Birth trauma,congenital malformations, and infections can increase the risk of epilepsy in this age group.

Children: The first year of life is a peak period for new cases of epilepsy, and the rate remains elevated until around age 10.

Older adults: After age 55, the risk of epilepsy rises again due to conditions like strokes, brain tumors, and Alzheimer's disease.

Other factors:

Family history: People with a family history of epilepsy are more likely to develop it themselves, although the risk is still relatively low.

Brain injuries: Head trauma, including concussions, can increase the risk of epilepsy.

Stroke: Strokes can damage brain tissue and lead to epilepsy.

Infections: Certain infections, such as meningitis, can also damage the brain and cause epilepsy.

Congenital malformations: Some people are born with malformations in their brains that make them more prone to seizures.

Metabolic imbalances: Conditions like diabetes and hypoglycemia can sometimes lead to seizures and epilepsy.

What occurs in the brain of an epileptic

The brain communicates through electrical signals between neurons. During a seizure, this normal electrical activity becomes disrupted, leading to abnormal and excessive electrical discharges.

Neurons, which are the basic building blocks of the brain, communicate by sending electrical signals through synapses, the junctions between neurons. These signals are carefully regulated to maintain the balance of electrical activity in the brain. In individuals with epilepsy, this balance is disturbed, and neurons may fire excessively, leading to a surge of electrical activity.

The brain can be compared to an intricate electrical circuit, and when the normal flow of electrical impulses is disrupted, it can result in a seizure. The abnormal electrical discharges can spread throughout the brain, causing various symptoms depending on the area affected. These symptoms can range from momentary lapses in awareness to more severe convulsions and loss of consciousness.

What occurs in the brain of an epileptic

affects not only the individual experiencing them but also ripples outward to impact their families in profound ways. The impact manifests on both physical and emotional levels, creating a tapestry of challenges and adaptations.

For individuals with epilepsy:

The fear and uncertainty of seizures: The unpredictable nature of seizures can cast a long shadow, causing anxiety and a constant awareness of vulnerability. This can limit social interactions, restrict independence, and hinder pursuit of opportunities.

Physical effects: The nature and frequency of seizures can lead to injuries,fatigue, and cognitive difficulties. Some types of medications can have side effects that further diminish well-being.

Stigma and discrimination: Misconceptions about epilepsy unfortunately persist, leading to social isolation, bullying, and limitations in career advancement. This stigma can be deeply damaging to self-esteem and mental health.

Psychological burden: Depression,anxiety, and low self-worth are common companions for individuals with epilepsy,further exacerbated by the challenges mentioned above. Managing these emotional effects is crucial for overall well-being.

For families:

The constant worry and fear: Witnessing seizures and the unpredictability they bring can be incredibly stressful for family members. The responsibility of caregiving,administering medication, and maintaining safety adds layers of burden.

Emotional turmoil: Guilt, helplessness, and frustration are common emotions experienced by family members, often intertwined with a desire to protect and shield the individual with epilepsy.

Social and financial strain: Epilepsy can disrupt family routines, limit social activities, and necessitate financial adjustments due to medical needs and potential employment limitations.

Disruptions in family dynamics: Roles and responsibilities within the family might shift, potentially causing resentment or frustration. Open communication and support are crucial to maintain a healthy family atmosphere.

Chapter 2

Types of Seizures

Common types of seizures and their characteristics

Healthcare providers classify epilepsies by their seizure type. Seizure categories are based on where they start in your brain, your level of awareness during a seizure and by presence or absence of muscle movements.

There are two major seizure groups:

Seizures with focal onset

One region, or network of cells, on one side of the brain is where focal onset seizures begin. There once was a term for this seizure: partial onset seizure. Two categories of focal seizures exist:

In a focal onset aware seizure, you are conscious and awake at the time of the seizure. Medical professionals used to refer to this as a straightforward partial seizure. Among the symptoms could be:

- alterations in the way that objects taste, smell, or sound.
- emotional shifts.
- jerking uncontrollably in the arms or legs.
- getting tingling, feeling lightheaded, and seeing flashing lights.

Seizures with focal onset reduced awareness

Indicates that you are disoriented or that you lost consciousness or awareness during the seizure. This kind of seizure was once known as a complicated partial seizure. Among the symptoms could be:

- A vacant gaze, or "staring into space."
- repetitive motions with the hand or fingers, such as rubbing, biting, or blinking of the eyes.

seizures of a generalized onset

Seizures with general onset simultaneously affect a large network of cells on both sides of your brain. There are six kinds of summed up seizures.

Non Appearance seizures: This seizure type causes a clear gaze or "gazing into space" (a concise loss of mindfulness). There might be minor muscle developments, including eye squinting, lip-smacking or biting movements, hand movements or scouring fingers. Absence seizures, which typically last less than ten seconds and are more prevalent in children, are frequently mistaken for daydreaming. This seizure type used to be called petit mal seizures.

Atonic seizures: Atonic signifies "without tone." When you have an atonic seizure, either your muscles are weak or you have lost muscle control. Portions of your body might hang or drop like your eyelids or head, or you might tumble to the ground during this short seizure (normally under 15 seconds). This seizure type is at times called "drop seizure" or "drop assault."

Epileptic fits: Tonic signifies "with tone." A tonic seizure implies your muscle tone has enormously expanded. You may fall because you are tense or stiff in your arms, legs, back, or entire body. You might know or have a little change in mindfulness during this short seizure (typically under 20 seconds).

Clonic seizures: " Clonus' ' signifies quick, continuing hardening and unwinding of a muscle ("jolting"). A clonic seizure happens when muscles constantly jerk for seconds to a moment or muscles solidify followed by jolting for seconds as long as two minutes.

Seizures with tinnitus: This seizure type is a blend of muscle solidness (tonic) and rehashed, cadenced muscle jolting (clonic). Medical services suppliers might call this seizure a spasm, and when called it an excellent mal seizure. Tonic-clonic seizures are a great many people's thought process when they hear "seizure." You black out, tumble to the ground, your muscles solidify and jolt for one to five minutes. You might poop or pee, bite your tongue, lose muscle control of your bowels or bladder, or drool.

Myoclonic seizures: This seizure type causes brief, shock-like muscle jerks or jerks ("myo" signifies muscle, "clonus" signifies muscle jolting). Myoclonic seizures generally last two or three seconds.

What causes seizures

Seizure triggers are occasions or something that occurs before the beginning of your seizure.

The following are common causes of seizures:

- Stress.
- Rest issues, for example, not resting soundly, not getting sufficient rest, being overtired, upset endlessly rest problems like rest apnea.
- Liquor use, liquor withdrawal, sporting medication use.
- Hormonal changes or feminine hormonal changes.
- Ailment, fever.
- Blazing lights or examples.
- Not practicing good eating habits, adjusted feasts or drinking an adequate number of liquids; nutrient and mineral insufficiencies, skipping dinners.
- Actual overexertion.
- Explicit food sources (caffeine is a typical trigger).
- Dehydration.
- a specific time of day or night.

- Utilization of specific drugs. A reported trigger is diphenhydramine, a component of over-the-counter remedies for colds, allergies, and insomnia.
- missed medication doses for seizures.

How can I identify the things that make me have seizures

Certain individuals find that their seizures happen reliably during specific times or around specific occasions or different elements. To see if there is a pattern, you might want to keep track of your seizures and the events that occur around them.

In your seizure journal, note the hour of day every seizure occurred, the occasions or extraordinary conditions occurring around the hour of the seizure and how you felt. Assuming that you suspect you've distinguished a trigger, track that trigger to see whether it's actually a trigger. For instance, on the off chance that you think caffeine is a seizure trigger, do you have a seizure in the wake of eating each juiced food or refreshment, later "x" number of

energized food sources/drinks or at specific
seasons of day subsequent to polishing off
caffeine? Caffeine might be the trigger when
completely looked into.

Chapter 3

Causes and Triggers of Epilepsy

Why people get epilepsy

In a majority of cases, up to 70%, the origin of seizures remains unknown. Recognized triggers encompass various factors, including:

Genetics: A few kinds of epilepsy (like adolescent myoclonic epilepsy and youth nonattendance epilepsy) are bound to run in families (acquired). That's what analysts trust in spite of the fact that there's some proof that particular qualities are involved, the qualities just increase the gamble of epilepsy, and different variables might be involved. There are sure epilepsies that outcome from irregularities that influence how synapses can speak with one another and can prompt unusual mind cues and seizures.

Mesial worldly sclerosis: This is a scar that structures in the internal piece of your transient curve (some portion of your mind close to your ear) that can lead to central seizures.

Head wounds: Head wounds can result from vehicular mishaps, falls or any hit to the head.

Mind diseases: Contaminations can incorporate mind ulcer, meningitis, encephalitis and neurocysticercosis.

autoimmune diseases Conditions that make your safe framework assault synapses (additionally called immune system infections) can prompt epilepsy.

Formative issues: Birth irregularities influencing the mind are a successive reason for epilepsy, especially in individuals whose seizures aren't controlled with hostile to seizure prescriptions. Some birth anomalies known to cause epilepsy incorporate central cortical dysplasia, polymicrogyria and tuberous sclerosis. Epilepsy can be brought on by a wide range of other brain abnormalities.

metabolic conditions: Individuals with a metabolic condition (how your body gets energy for typical capabilities) can have epilepsy. Your medical care supplier can identify a considerable lot of these problems through hereditary tests.

Anomalies of the brain's blood vessels and conditions. Cerebrum medical problems that can cause epilepsy incorporate mind growths, strokes, dementia and unusual veins, like arteriovenous distortions.

Exploring common triggers and how to manage them

Exploring common triggers of seizures and understanding how to manage them is crucial for individuals dealing with epilepsy. Let's delve into this topic by breaking it down into simpler terms.

Sleep Deprivation:
Explanation: Lack of proper sleep can be a significant trigger for seizures.
Management: Ensure a consistent sleep schedule, prioritize quality sleep, and create a relaxing bedtime routine.

Stress and Anxiety:

Explanation: Emotional stress and anxiety can contribute to seizure activity.
Management: Practice stress-reducing techniques like deep breathing, meditation, and mindfulness. Regular exercise can also be beneficial.

Explanation: Irregular or missed doses of prescribed medications can disrupt seizure control.
Management: Establish a medication routine, set alarms, use pill organizers, and communicate openly with healthcare providers about any challenges.

Fluctuations in Medication Levels:
Explanation: Abrupt changes in medication levels can trigger seizures.
Management: Strictly follow the prescribed dosage, consult with healthcare professionals before any adjustments, and report any side effects promptly.

Alcohol and Substance Use:
Explanation: Excessive alcohol consumption and certain substances can lower the seizure threshold.
Management: Limit or avoid alcohol and illicit substances. Inform healthcare providers about any prescribed medications to assess potential interactions.

Lack of Routine:

Explanation: Disruptions to daily routines can impact seizure control.

Management: Establish and maintain a consistent daily schedule. Predictability can be beneficial in managing seizures.

Flashing Lights (Photosensitivity):

Explanation: Some individuals with epilepsy are sensitive to flashing lights.

Management: Identify and avoid triggers such as strobe lights or video games with rapid flashing. Use precautions, like wearing sunglasses in bright environments.

Hormonal Changes:

Explanation: Hormonal fluctuations, especially in women, can influence seizure activity.

Management: Women should work closely with healthcare providers to manage hormonal changes, particularly during menstruation.

Chapter 4

Diagnosis and Treatment

Navigating the diagnostic process

Navigating the diagnostic process of epilepsy is a multifaceted journey that involves various medical assessments and examinations. Let's unravel this process, simplifying the complexities for a clearer understanding.

Clinical History:

Explanation: The initial step involves a thorough discussion about the individual's medical history, including any previous seizures, associated symptoms, and potential triggers.
Understanding: Doctors ask questions to gather information about the nature, frequency, and circumstances surrounding seizures, helping to establish a baseline for diagnosis.

Physical Examination:

Explanation: A comprehensive physical examination is conducted to identify any neurological signs or abnormalities.

Understanding: Doctors assess reflexes, muscle strength, and coordination, looking for physical indicators that may be linked to epilepsy.

Diagnostic Tests:

Explanation: Various tests may be recommended to aid in the diagnosis.

Understanding: This can include an Electroencephalogram (EEG), which measures brain waves, and imaging studies such as Magnetic Resonance Imaging (MRI) or Computed Tomography (CT) scans, providing detailed pictures of the brain.

Blood Tests:

Explanation: Blood tests may be conducted to rule out other medical conditions that could be causing seizures.

Understanding: These tests help ensure a comprehensive evaluation, eliminating potential underlying factors beyond epilepsy.

Video EEG Monitoring:

Explanation: In some cases, individuals may undergo video EEG monitoring, where they are observed while connected to an EEG for an extended period.

Understanding: This helps capture and analyze real-time brain activity during seizures, aiding in a more precise diagnosis.

Provocative Testing:

Explanation: Occasionally, doctors may use specific triggers during EEG monitoring to provoke seizures for a more accurate diagnosis.

Understanding: This controlled environment helps healthcare professionals observe and analyze seizure patterns, contributing to a more tailored treatment plan.

Collaboration with Specialists:

Explanation: Neurologists often collaborate with other specialists, such as epileptologists, to ensure a comprehensive evaluation.

Understanding: This multidisciplinary approach ensures that all aspects of the diagnostic process are thoroughly explored, offering a more accurate diagnosis and personalized care.

Patient Education:

Explanation: Throughout the diagnostic process, patients and their families are educated about epilepsy, potential triggers, and available treatment options.

Understanding: This empowers individuals to actively participate in their healthcare, fostering a collaborative approach between patients and healthcare providers.

The diagnosis of epilepsy

Diagnosing epilepsy involves a comprehensive process that combines medical history, clinical evaluations, and diagnostic tests. Let's break down this complex journey into simpler terms for a better understanding.

Medical History:

Explanation: The first step involves discussing the individual's medical history with a healthcare professional.

Process: The doctor will inquire about past seizures, their frequency, duration, and any potential triggers. Information about family history, overall health, and medications is also collected.

Clinical Evaluation:

Explanation: A thorough physical and neurological examination is conducted.
Process: The healthcare provider assesses the individual's overall health and performs neurological tests to check reflexes, muscle tone, and coordination. This helps in identifying any signs of neurological abnormalities.

Electroencephalogram (EEG):

Explanation: An EEG is a key tool in epilepsy diagnosis, measuring electrical activity in the brain.
Process: Electrodes are placed on the scalp to record brain waves. Patterns indicative of epilepsy, such as abnormal spikes or sharp waves, can be observed. Sometimes, prolonged EEG monitoring (24-hour or more) may be necessary for a comprehensive assessment.

Imaging Studies:

Explanation: Imaging tests like MRI and CT scans are conducted to identify any structural abnormalities in the brain.
Process: These scans provide detailed images of the brain's structure, helping to identify tumors, lesions, or other issues that may contribute to seizures.

Blood Tests:

Explanation: Blood tests are performed to rule out underlying medical conditions.
Process: The analysis helps detect conditions such as metabolic disorders, infections, or genetic factors that may be associated with seizures.

Additional Tests:

Explanation: In some cases, additional specialized tests may be recommended.
Examples: Video EEG monitoring, which records both brain activity and the individual's behavior during seizures, or neuropsychological tests to assess cognitive function.

Collaboration and Follow-up:

Explanation: Diagnosis often involves collaboration between healthcare professionals.
Process: Neurologists, epilepsy specialists, and other healthcare providers work together to interpret test results and reach a conclusive diagnosis. Regular follow-ups are essential to monitor progress, adjust treatment plans, and address any concerns.

Medications

Epilepsy, a neurological condition causing seizures, can be effectively managed with medication. But navigating the world of epilepsy drugs can feel like deciphering a foreign language. Let's break it down to simpler terms, making you feel more informed and empowered about your treatment journey.

Imagine your brain as a bustling city:

Neurons: These are the citizens, sending and receiving messages through electrical signals.

Neurotransmitters: Think of them as mail carriers, delivering chemical messages between neurons.

Seizures: When the electrical activity goes haywire, it's like a traffic jam, causing abnormal signals and symptoms like uncontrolled movements or loss of consciousness.

Epilepsy medication:

Traffic cops: These drugs work by regulating the electrical activity in the brain, calming down overexcited neurons and preventing traffic jams.

Different types of cops: Just like there are different types of traffic police, there are various classes of epilepsy drugs, each targeting different neurotransmitters and mechanisms.

Here are the main types of epilepsy medications:

Sodium channel blockers: These are like stop signs, slowing down the firing of neurons and preventing them from getting too excited. Examples include carbamazepine, oxcarbazepine, and lamotrigine.

Calcium channel blockers: These act like roadblocks, hindering the flow of calcium into neurons, which is needed for them to fire. Examples include ethosuximide and zonisamide.

GABAergic drugs: These mimic the action of a calming neurotransmitter called GABA, quieting down overactive neurons.Examples include gabapentin,phenobarbital, and valproic acid.

Choosing the right medication:

It's like finding the right traffic solution for your specific city. Your doctor will consider the type of seizures you have, your medical history, and other factors to choose the most effective and safe medication for you.

It's a journey, not a destination. Finding the right medication may take time and adjustments. Be patient, communicate openly with your doctor, and don't hesitate to ask questions.

Alternative therapies

Epilepsy, a neurological condition causing seizures, can be effectively managed with traditional medication. But for some, exploring alternative therapies alongside mainstream treatment offers a holistic approach to well-being. Let's delve into some of these options, explained in a way even your friendly neighborhood baker can understand!

Mind-Body Magic:

Yoga and Meditation: Imagine your brain as a bustling marketplace. Yoga and meditation are like deep breaths, calming the chaos and promoting inner peace. This can reduce stress, a common seizure trigger, and improve overall well-being. Think of it as decluttering your mental space for smoother brain traffic flow.

Biofeedback: This is like a brain game where you learn to control your body's responses. Imagine flashing lights reflecting your brainwaves. Biofeedback helps you "train" your brain to stay calm, potentially reducing seizure frequency. It's like teaching your brain to sing a soothing tune instead of a chaotic rock ballad.

Dietary Delights:

Ketogenic Diet: Ditch the carbs, embrace the fats! This high-fat, low-carb diet mimics the metabolic state of fasting, which can have anti-seizure effects. Think of it as giving your brain a different kind of fuel, sometimes leading to smoother engine operation (your brain, in this case!).

Modified Atkins Diet: Similar to keto, this diet restricts carbs but allows for more protein and some vegetables. It's like taking the keto highway with a scenic detour through veggie land.

Natural Helpers:

CBD Oil: A cannabis-derived compound, CBD oil has shown promise in reducing seizure frequency in some types of epilepsy. Think of it as a natural calming agent, like a gentle nudge towards brain serenity.

Melatonin: This sleep hormone can also help regulate brain activity and potentially reduce seizures. Imagine it as a bedtime lullaby for your brain, promoting restful sleep and potentially calmer mornings.

Choosing the right treatment plan for you

Epilepsy, with its unpredictable seizures, can feel like a storm cloud looming over daily life. But amidst the uncertainty, there's hope. Finding the right treatment plan is like charting a course through the storm, guiding you towards calmer seas and a brighter future. This guide equips you with the knowledge and resources to navigate this journey with confidence.

Step 1: Understanding Your Epilepsy

Every epilepsy journey is unique. The first step is uncovering the specifics of yours:

Seizure types: Recognizing the different types of seizures you experience is crucial.Think of them as unique weather patterns in your brain's storm system.

Seizure triggers: Identifying what triggers your seizures, like stress or lack of sleep, is like pinpointing the storm's brewing grounds.

Underlying cause: If there's an underlying cause, like a brain tumor, addressing it might be the key to calming the storm altogether.

Step 2: Exploring Treatment Options

The treatment toolbox for epilepsy is diverse, offering options to fit various needs:

Medication: The mainstay of epilepsy treatment, medications work by regulating brain activity and preventing seizures. Think of them as weatherproofing your brain against the storm.

Diet therapy: Specific diets like ketogenic or modified Atkins can alter brain metabolism and potentially reduce seizures. Imagine modifying the storm's fuel source to weaken its intensity.

Brain stimulation therapies: Techniques like vagus nerve stimulation or deep brain stimulation send electrical impulses to regulate brain activity. Think of them as gentle nudges to guide the storm towards calmer waters.

Surgery: In some cases, surgery to remove the seizure-causing area of the brain might be an option. Imagine it as strategically plucking the storm's eye to weaken its overall power.

Step 3: Partnering with Your Healthcare Team

Choosing the right treatment is a collaborative effort. Your healthcare team, including neurologists, epilepsy specialists, and therapists, will guide you through your options, considering your specific needs and preferences. Think of them as your experienced navigators, helping you choose the optimal route through the storm.

Part 2: Living Well with Epilepsy

Chapter 5

Managing Medication

Understanding medication types and side effects

with the wide range of available medications, understanding their types and potential side effects is essential for informed decision-making.

Medication Types:

Anti-seizure medications (ASMs): These are the primary medications used to prevent seizures. They work by targeting different mechanisms in the brain to modulate neuronal activity and suppress abnormal electrical discharges. Some common ASM types include:

- Sodium channel blockers:Carbamazepine, Oxcarbazepine,Lamotrigine
- Calcium channel blockers:Ethosuximide, Zonisamide
- GABAergic drugs: Levetiracetam,Valproic acid, Topiramate

- Benzodiazepines: Clonazepam,Diazepam
  (primarily used for rescue in emergencies)

Other medications: Depending on the underlying cause of epilepsy or the presence of comorbidities, other medications might be prescribed to manage specific symptoms, such as:

- Antidepressants: For managing depression or anxiety commonly associated with epilepsy
- Pain medications: For pain associated with specific epilepsy syndromes
- Hormonal therapy: For women with epilepsy affected by menstrual cycles

Side Effects:

Like all medications, ASMs can have side effects. The severity and type of side effects vary depending on the specific medication, dosage, and individual factors. Some common side effects include:

- Drowsiness or fatigue
- Dizziness or balance problems
- Cognitive issues: memory problems, difficulty concentrating
- Nausea, vomiting, or stomach upset
- Headaches
- Skin rashes
- Mood changes (anxiety, depression)
- Weight gain or loss
- Hair loss
- Birth defects (for some medications)

Managing Side Effects:

Open communication with your doctor: Discussing concerns and side effects openly with your doctor is crucial. They can adjust the dosage, switch medications,or suggest alternative management strategies.

Starting with low doses: Often, starting with a low dose and gradually increasing it can help minimize side effects.

Treating specific side effects: Some side effects, like nausea or headaches, can be managed with additional medications.

Non-pharmacological approaches: Maintaining a healthy lifestyle, including regular sleep, exercise, and balanced diet,can contribute to managing side effects and overall well-being.

Tips for medication adherence and avoiding missed doses

 Managing epilepsy often revolves around medication, and consistently taking your doses as prescribed is paramount. But let's face it, life throws curveballs, and missed doses happen. The good news? You can conquer the "missed dose monster" with some strategic tips and tricks.

Mastering the Routine:

Schedule it up: Set alarms, reminders, or notifications on your phone or pill dispenser to nudge you at medication times.

Link it to habits: Take your meds alongside routine actions like brushing your teeth or making coffee.

Find your groove: Experiment with different dosing times to find what fits your day (morning, bedtime, after meals?).

Prepare for travel: Pack medications in convenient travel containers and refill prescriptions before trips.

Outsmarting the Obstacles:

Simplify your regimen: Talk to your doctor about simplifying your dosage schedule or using long-acting medications if possible.

Befriend medication tracking apps: Utilize apps to log doses, set reminders, and track progress.

Enlist your support team: Share your challenges with family, friends, or healthcare professionals. *Their encouragement and accountability can be invaluable.*

Address side effects: If side effects are making adherence difficult, discuss them with your doctor. Adjustments or alternative medications might be possible.

Beyond the Pills:

Understand the "why": Knowing how your medication works and its importance in seizure control can boost motivation.

Celebrate your wins: Reward yourself for consistent adherence, even with small milestones.

Embrace open communication: Talk to your doctor openly about any difficulties or concerns you have about taking your medication.

Chapter 6

Lifestyle and Self-Care

Maintaining a healthy diet and exercise routine

Maintaining a healthy diet and exercise routine is vital for individuals with epilepsy, as it can positively impact overall well-being and potentially contribute to better seizure control. Let's break down these aspects in a way that's easily understandable.

Diet for Epilepsy:

Balanced Nutrition: Focus on a balanced diet that includes a variety of foods, providing essential nutrients like vitamins and minerals. This helps support overall health and may contribute to better seizure management.

Ketogenic Diet:

Some individuals with epilepsy find success with a ketogenic diet, which is high in fats, moderate in proteins, and low in carbohydrates. This diet mimics the metabolic state of fasting and may help reduce seizures in some cases.

Hydration:Stay adequately hydrated.

Dehydration can affect medication levels and potentially trigger seizures, so it's crucial to maintain a regular intake of water throughout the day.

Exercise for Epilepsy:

Regular Physical Activity: Engage in regular, moderate-intensity exercise. This can include activities like walking, swimming, or cycling. Exercise not only promotes overall health but also contributes to stress reduction, a common trigger for seizures.

Routine and Consistency: Establish a consistent exercise routine. Regularity in physical activity helps in maintaining overall fitness and may contribute to a more stable mood, positively impacting seizure thresholds.

Considerations for Layman Understanding:

Consultation with Healthcare Team: Always consult with your healthcare team before making significant changes to your diet or exercise routine. They can provide guidance tailored to your specific health needs and any potential interactions with medications.

Gradual Changes: Make changes gradually. Whether adjusting your diet or starting a new exercise routine, small and gradual changes are often more sustainable and easier to adapt to.

Listen to Your Body: Pay attention to how your body responds. If you notice any adverse effects or changes in seizure patterns, communicate promptly with your healthcare team. This ensures timely adjustments to your plan.

Mind-Body Connection: Recognize the mind-body connection. Practices like yoga or meditation can complement your routine by promoting relaxation and stress reduction.

Community Support: Join epilepsy support groups or communities. Sharing experiences and tips with others who have epilepsy can provide valuable insights and encouragement.

Getting enough sleep and managing stress

Epilepsy, a neurological condition characterized by recurrent seizures, affects millions worldwide. While medication plays a crucial role in managing seizures, two often-overlooked lifestyle factors can significantly impact your well-being and seizure control: sleep and stress. Getting enough restful sleep and managing stress effectively are like sturdy pillars supporting your epilepsy management plan. Let's explore how these pillars work together for a healthier, happier you.

The Sweet Symphony of Sleep:

Sleep and Seizures: Imagine your brain as a bustling orchestra. When you're well-rested, the instruments play in harmony, producing beautiful music. But sleep deprivation is like a conductor losing control, leading to discord and potentially triggering seizures. Studies show a clear link between sleep deprivation and increased seizure frequency and severity.

The Restorative Power: During sleep, your brain goes through essential maintenance processes, clearing harmful toxins and strengthening neural connections. This nightly tune-up is crucial for optimal brain function and seizure control. Aim for 7-8 hours of quality sleep each night to keep your brain's orchestra in perfect harmony.

Stress: The Unwelcome Guest:

Stress and Seizures: Chronic stress can be like an unwelcome guest at your brain's party, throwing the mood off and potentially triggering seizures. Stress hormones like cortisol can disrupt brain activity and lower the seizure threshold, making you more susceptible to attacks.

Calming the Chaos: Finding healthy ways to manage stress is essential for epilepsy management. Activities like yoga, meditation, deep breathing exercises, and spending time in nature can help quiet the storm within and promote relaxation. Remember, a calm mind translates to a calmer brain, reducing the risk of seizures.

Weaving the Pillars Together:

Lifestyle Harmony: Think of sleep and stress management as threads woven into the fabric of your epilepsy management plan. By prioritizing both adequate sleep and healthy stress-coping mechanisms, you create a stronger, more resilient tapestry of well-being.

Working with Your Doctor: Discuss your sleep and stress concerns with your doctor. They can offer personalized advice and recommend strategies to optimize your sleep hygiene and manage stress effectively. Remember, a collaborative approach is key to success.

Sweet Dreams, Less Stress, Fewer Seizures:

By prioritizing sleep and stress management alongside your medication regimen, you empower yourself to take control of your epilepsy and pave the way for a healthier, happier future.

Building a support system and coping with emotional challenges

Amidst the storm, building a strong support system and developing effective coping mechanisms can be the anchors that keep you afloat. Imagine it as constructing a sanctuary – a safe haven where you can find understanding, strength, and the courage to navigate the emotional challenges of epilepsy.

Building Your Support Team:

The foundation of your sanctuary is a diverse and dedicated support team. Think of them as pillars, each offering unique strength and perspective.

Medical Professionals: Neurologists, epilepsy specialists, and therapists are your frontline, providing medical guidance, personalized treatment plans, and emotional support.

Family and Friends: Your closest circle offers unconditional love, understanding, and practical help. Share openly about your needs and invite them to learn more about epilepsy.

Support Groups: Connecting with others living with epilepsy provides a sense of belonging and shared experiences. You can find in-person or online groups to offer and receive support, tips, and empathy.

Therapists: A therapist can be a confidential space to explore emotional challenges like anxiety, depression, and frustration. They can equip you with coping mechanisms and strategies to manage stress and build resilience.

Passionate Advocates: Consider engaging with epilepsy advocacy groups or organizations. By raising awareness and promoting understanding, you empower both yourself and others living with the condition.

Qualities of a Strong Support Team Player:

Not everyone is suited to be a pillar in your sanctuary. Look for individuals who possess these qualities:

Active Listening: They provide a safe space for you to express your fears, frustrations, and triumphs without judgment.

Empathy and Understanding: They make a genuine effort to understand your journey and the challenges you face.

Patience and Acceptance: They respect your individuality and the time it takes to adjust to living with epilepsy.

Positivity and Encouragement: They offer words of affirmation and celebrate your successes, big and small.

Reliability and Consistency: They show up consistently and offer unwavering support, even when things get tough.

Chapter 6

Safety and Everyday Activities

Driving, working, and participating in daily activities

Epilepsy affects over 50 million people worldwide, and living with seizures can present unique challenges in everyday life, including driving, working, and participating in daily activities. However, with proper precautions and education, people with epilepsy can live fulfilling and independent lives. **Here are some safety tips for navigating these areas:**

Driving:

Follow doctor's advice: Adhere to your doctor's recommendations regarding driving restrictions based on your seizure type and frequency.

Maintain seizure control: Optimize your seizure control through medication, lifestyle changes, and regular doctor visits.

Inform licensing authorities: Report your epilepsy diagnosis to the relevant licensing authorities as required by law.

Carry emergency information: Always carry a MedicAlert bracelet or card with updated medical information.

Plan ahead: Avoid driving when tired, stressed, or experiencing seizure warning signs.

Prioritize passenger safety: Consider having a driving buddy if your seizures are unpredictable.

Working:

Open communication: Discuss your epilepsy with your employer in a confidential setting.

Accommodations: Work collaboratively with your employer to identify and implement reasonable accommodations, such as flexible scheduling or modified tasks.

Emergency plan: Develop a workplace seizure action plan with colleagues and supervisors.

Know your rights: Familiarize yourself with disability discrimination laws and resources.

Focus on strengths: Highlight your skills and abilities, and contribute meaningfully to your workplace.

Daily Activities:

Identify triggers: Be aware of factors that might trigger your seizures, such as sleep deprivation, stress, or flashing lights.

Maintain a healthy lifestyle: Prioritize regular sleep, a balanced diet, and physical exercise to manage stress and promote overall well-being.

Plan and prepare: Take preventative measures before engaging in activities that pose potential risks, such as swimming alone or using cooking appliances.

Wear protective gear: Consider using helmets for cycling, knee pads for falls, and other safety equipment as needed.

Communicate with loved ones: Educate family and friends about epilepsy and your specific needs.

Seek support: Connect with epilepsy support groups or online communities for understanding, resources, and encouragement.

Travel tips for individuals with epilepsy

Traveling with epilepsy requires some extra planning and preparation, but it doesn't have to hold you back from exploring the world! Here are some tips to ensure a safe and enjoyable trip:

Before you go:

Consult your doctor: Discuss your travel plans with your doctor well in advance. They can assess your seizure risk, adjust medications if needed, and provide a letter explaining your condition for emergencies.

Pack smart: Pack enough medication for the entire trip, plus at least a few extra doses in case of delays. Keep medications in their original containers and in your carry-on luggage. Pack a first-aid kit with any necessary medical supplies.

Research your destination: Find out about healthcare facilities near your accommodation, local emergency numbers, and accessibility options. Check if your epilepsy medications are available in your destination country.

Consider travel insurance: Invest in travel insurance that covers medical emergencies and unexpected delays.

Inform travel companions: Tell your travel partners about your epilepsy, what to do in case of a seizure, and how to contact your emergency contacts.

Wear medical ID: Consider wearing a medical ID bracelet or carrying an epilepsy ID card. This can provide information to others in case of an emergency.

While traveling:

Prioritize sleep and stress management: Lack of sleep and stress can trigger seizures. Stick to your regular sleep schedule as much as possible and incorporate relaxation techniques like meditation or deep breathing.
Stay hydrated and well-nourished: Dehydration and electrolyte imbalance can contribute to seizures. Drink plenty of water, eat regular meals, and avoid excessive alcohol and caffeine.
Be mindful of triggers: Identify your personal seizure triggers, such as flashing lights, loud

noises, or extreme temperatures, and avoid them as much as possible.

Take breaks and listen to your body: Traveling can be tiring. Plan frequent breaks, delegate tasks, and adjust your itinerary if needed. Don't push yourself too hard.

Inform airline or travel service providers: If flying, inform the airline about your epilepsy. You may be able to request an aisle seat or other accommodations. If taking a cruise or tour, inform the provider in advance.

Carry emergency contact information: Keep a list of emergency contact numbers readily available, including your doctor, local healthcare facilities, and family/friends.

Additional Tips:

- Consider wearing comfortable clothing and shoes that are easy to remove in case of a seizure.
- Pack a small notebook or journal to record your daily experiences and track your epilepsy triggers.
- Connect with epilepsy communities online or in your destination city for support and advice.

- Focus on having fun and enjoying your trip! Remember, epilepsy doesn't have to define your travel experiences.

Planning for the future and managing life transitions

Living with epilepsy can come with its own set of challenges, and navigating life transitions can be particularly daunting. However, with careful planning and proactive management, individuals with epilepsy can confidently embrace new opportunities and ensure their well-being throughout their life journey. Here are some key considerations for planning the future and managing life transitions:

Education and Self-Awareness:

Understanding your epilepsy: The first step is to gain a comprehensive understanding of your specific type of epilepsy, triggers, and effective seizure management strategies. This knowledge empowers you to make informed decisions about your future and advocate for your needs.

Communicating with healthcare professionals: Maintain open communication with your neurologist and other healthcare providers. Discuss your future plans and any concerns you have about transitions. They can provide guidance and tailor treatment plans to support your goals.

Staying informed about advancements: Keep yourself updated on the latest research and developments in epilepsy treatment and management. This knowledge can help you make informed choices and advocate for yourself in various settings.

Planning for Education and Employment:

Academic Success: Discuss your epilepsy with educators and disability services to ensure you have access to necessary accommodations and support to excel in your studies.
Career Choices: Explore career options that align with your interests and abilities while considering potential seizure triggers and safety factors. Networking with professionals with epilepsy can offer valuable insights and encouragement.

Disability Rights and Advocacy: Understand your rights under disability laws and regulations in your region. This knowledge empowers you to advocate for fair treatment and accommodations in educational and professional settings.

Building a Support System:

Family and Friends: Openly communicate your epilepsy with your loved ones and involve them in your planning process. Their understanding and support can be invaluable during transitions.

Support Groups and Organizations: Connect with communities and organizations dedicated to supporting people with epilepsy. Sharing experiences and learning from others can provide valuable guidance and encouragement.

Mental Health Support: Managing life transitions can be stressful. Consider seeking mental health support from a therapist or counselor specializing in epilepsy to navigate challenges and build resilience.

Financial Planning and Stability:

Understanding Insurance and Benefits:
Familiarize yourself with your health insurance
coverage and any disability benefits you may be
eligible for. This will help you plan for future
healthcare needs and secure financial stability.
Employment and Income Security: Explore
options for financial stability, including employment
opportunities, disability benefits, and government
assistance programs.
Emergency Preparedness: Develop a plan for
managing your epilepsy in case of emergencies or
unexpected situations. This includes having a
seizure action plan, emergency contact information
readily available, and ensuring access to
medication.

Maintaining Emotional and Physical
Well-being:

Prioritize Self-Care: Invest in activities that
promote your emotional and physical well-being,
such as regular exercise, healthy eating habits, and
stress management techniques. These practices
can contribute to overall health and resilience
during life transitions.
Positive Mindset and Resilience: Cultivate a
positive outlook and develop coping strategies to
manage stress and challenges. Remember, life

transitions are natural, and with proactive planning and support, you can navigate them successfully while living well with epilepsy.

Note: Planning for the future and managing life transitions is an ongoing process. Be adaptable, seek support when needed, and celebrate your achievements along the way. With dedication and resilience, you can build a fulfilling life and embrace new opportunities while living with epilepsy.

10 DAYS MEAL PLAN.

Meal 1: Breakfast - Keto Omelette

Ingredients: Eggs, spinach, feta cheese, olive oil

How to make: Whisk eggs, sauté spinach in olive oil, add eggs, and top with feta.

Meal 2: Snack - Avocado and Bacon

Ingredients: Avocado, bacon strips

How to make: Slice avocado, wrap with bacon, bake until crispy.

Meal 3: Lunch - Grilled Chicken Salad

Ingredients: Grilled chicken, mixed greens, cherry tomatoes, olive oil dressing

How to make: Grill chicken, toss with veggies, drizzle with olive oil dressing.

Meal 4: Snack - Greek Yogurt with Berries
Ingredients: Greek yogurt, mixed berries
How to make: Mix yogurt with berries for a protein-packed snack.

Meal 5: Dinner - Salmon with Broccoli
Ingredients: Salmon fillet, broccoli, lemon, herbs
How to make: Bake salmon with lemon and herbs, steam broccoli.

Meal 6: Snack - Cheese and Almonds
Ingredients: Cheese cubes, almonds
How to make: Pair cheese cubes with almonds for a satisfying snack.

Meal 7: Smoothie - Berry Keto Smoothie
Ingredients: Berries, almond milk, chia seeds, protein powder

How to make: Blend berries, almond milk, chia seeds, and protein powder.

Meal 8: Dessert - Dark Chocolate Avocado Mousse
Ingredients: Avocado, dark chocolate, vanilla extract
How to make: Blend avocado, melted chocolate, and vanilla for a creamy mousse.

Meal 9: Snack - Cucumber Slices with Hummus
Ingredients: Cucumber, hummus
How to make: Slice cucumber, serve with hummus.

Meal 10: Dinner - Zucchini Noodles with Pesto
Ingredients: Zucchini noodles, pesto sauce, grilled chicken

How to make: Spiralize zucchini, toss with pesto, and top with grilled chicken.

30 DAYS EXERCISE FOR YOU

Warm-up: Start with 5-10 minutes of light cardio (walking or cycling).
Stretching: Focus on major muscle groups, holding each stretch for 15-30 seconds.
Low-impact cardio: Engage in activities like swimming or stationary cycling for 20-30 minutes.
Impact: Improves cardiovascular health, reduces stress, and promotes overall well-being.

Day 6-10:

Strength training: Include bodyweight exercises like squats, lunges, and push-ups.
Core exercises: Planks and gentle abdominal exercises for 15-20 minutes.
Cool down: Finish with 5-10 minutes of light stretching.

Impact: Enhances muscle tone, supports joint health, and boosts metabolism.

Day 11-15:

Cardiovascular exercise: Increase intensity with brisk walking or jogging for 30 minutes.
Flexibility training: Incorporate yoga or Pilates for balance and flexibility.
Deep breathing exercises: Practice controlled breathing for 10 minutes.
Impact: Strengthens respiratory function, improves flexibility, and aids stress management.

Day 16-20:

Interval training: Alternate between bursts of high-intensity and low-intensity exercises.
Balance exercises: Include single-leg stands and stability exercises.
Relaxation techniques: Try meditation or mindfulness for 10-15 minutes.

Impact: Enhances cardiovascular fitness, improves balance, and reduces anxiety.

Day 21-25:

Moderate-intensity cardio: Engage in activities like brisk walking or cycling for 40 minutes.
Cross-training: Introduce a new activity to keep things interesting.
Progressive muscle relaxation: Release tension in muscles through systematic relaxation.
Impact: Boosts endurance, prevents exercise monotony, and promotes relaxation.

Day 26-30:

Full-body workout: Combine strength, cardio, and flexibility exercises.
Circuit training: Perform a series of exercises with minimal rest between sets.
Reflect and adjust: Evaluate progress, make necessary adjustments, and plan for continued exercise.

Impact: Achieves a balanced fitness routine, promotes adaptability, and supports long-term adherence.

Conclusion

In concluding "Beating Epilepsy: A Comprehensive Guide for Living Well with Epilepsy for Newly Diagnosed Patients and Caregivers," I want to emphasize the strength, resilience, and knowledge gained on this journey. Living with epilepsy poses challenges, but through understanding, support, and the strategies outlined in this guide, individuals and their caregivers can navigate this path with confidence.

Remember, you are not alone. This book aimed to provide insights, practical tips, and a sense of empowerment. Embrace the journey, celebrate small victories, and always prioritize your well-being. Beating epilepsy is not just about managing seizures; it's about leading a fulfilling life, and with the right tools and mindset, you can overcome obstacles and thrive. Wishing you a future filled with resilience, hope, and a life lived well beyond the constraints of epilepsy.